Table Of Contents

Table Of Contents

Introduction

Keep up to Date with New Releases

Chapter 1 Battling Acne with a Healthy Diet

Chapter 2 Eliminating Acne by Changing Your Lifestyle

Chapter 3 Comprehensive Anti-Acne Skin Care Regimen

Chapter 4 3 DIY Facial Scrubs

Chapter 5 15 Lush DIY Facial Masks

Chapter 6 Oil Pulling

Chapter 7 Clean Your Skin Like an Egyptian

Chapter 8 Getting Rid of Acne Scars

Chapter 8 Controlling Your Stress Levels

Steps to Success Action Plan

Conclusion

Bonus Chapter

Other Books you may be interested in...

Free Gift

Introduction

Are you sick of having ugly scars?

Sick of Yucky Pimples all the time?

Do you want firmer skin, softer skin, and younger skin?

Are you worried you'll never have gorgeous clear skin?

Are you sick of piling on layers of makeup to hide your face?

Do you look at magazines and just wish your skin was as beautiful and dewy as the other girls?

Do you look at yourself and find it hard to imagine having beautiful clear skin?

Do you wish you knew how to have clear skin for life?

Or maybe just for a night?

In this book you will discover the most up-to-date information on how to have clear skin and beat acne for life and the best ways do it including:

-What is acne?

-What type of acne do you have?

-Can diet really affect your skin?

-Does lifestyle affect your skin?

-A little known Skin Care Secret from the Egyptians

-The Benefits of Oil Pulling!

-3 All Natural facial scrubs

& 15 Lush All natural homemade facemask recipes

And much more!

I want to thank you and congratulate you for downloading the book, *Skin Care Secrets You Wish You Knew!* Taking the first step is sometimes half of the battle!

I would also like to introduce myself; my name is Simone, the creator of the Healthy Body Books. My deep-seated passion for health has driven me to create these books. Something inside of me has always called out, encouraging me to write books that health-minded individuals would want to read. Health has always been a priority in my life, even when a recent change in my routine made it much more difficult to find myself.

In spite of not feeling my best (or even much like myself), I found ways to continue achieving my goals. After searching long and hard, I found that natural therapies, diets and self-help were enough to help me get things back under control. I found out that these natural remedies were doing so much for me – and I never looked back.

If you are trying to find another way to stay healthy, the Healthy Body Books are for you. If you are anything like me, you might need to find an alternative method to reach your peak. Written by experts in terms that anybody can read, these books are designed to help you identify which aspects of your life just do not seem to be working for you. You should not let anything stop you from being the person you want to be – or from living the life you want to live. This book will help you along you journey.

Good luck!

Chapter 1 Battling Acne with a Healthy Diet

Millions of people worldwide suffer from acne. For many of us, this common skin problem is the bane of our existence. Medically known as Acne Vulgaris, acne typically occurs in teenage years but also persists even in adulthood. It doesn't happen to younger people only; adults can also suffer from acne.

What comprises acne? A pimple lies in the middle of an acne. It's known as a plug of keratin, skin debris and fat all stuck inside a hair duct. An open pimple is called a blackhead while a closed one is referred to as a whitehead. Usually, whiteheads cause ruptures in the walls of a hair duct, hence leading to infection, redness, pustules and cysts of acne.

Aside from poor hygiene, there are various factors that cause acne. Teens tend to experience acne breakouts due to fast hormonal and physical changes. Moreover, unhealthy diet and sleep deprivation also trigger acne breakouts.

If you've been struggling with acne and you haven't found the right solutions to treat this skin condition as of yet, this guide will help you completely get rid of it so you can finally attain your most desired flawless skin. It doesn't matter whether you're in your puberty phase or you're on the brink of adulthood already. There are certainly effective ways to eliminate acne and maintain a clear and smooth skin.

Have a Healthy Meal Plan for Acne-Free Skin

Consuming a healthy diet is crucial to maintaining clear, acne-free skin. Getting rid of acne is not just about tackling the problem outside; you also need to pay attention to what you feed your body in order to keep your skin clean, smooth and glowing. Maintaining a healthy diet will definitely bring numerous benefits to your body aside from eliminating acne.

Do you like to eat fruits and vegetables, or do you prefer to munch on junk foods and oily meals from fast-food restaurants? Check your diet and see if you eat starch-rich, fatty and sugary items more than healthy foods. You should know by now that junk foods are bad for your body in many ways. Acne tends to worsen because of bad eating habits. To beat acne for life, you need to focus on your everyday diet and make yourself healthier inside and out.

Remember: Skin health is strongly affected by your diet. People who eat healthy foods, especially fruits and vegetables, have lesser chances of getting acne mainly because these foods are rich in anti-inflammatory compounds and antioxidants.

So, the first step towards clearing up your skin is to watch your diet and develop a healthy meal plan.

The Best Diet Plan for Getting Rid of Acne

1. Foods Rich in Zinc – Most health professionals agree that zinc is a powerful mineral when it comes to fighting acne. Its primary role is to maintain a keen sense of smell, strengthen the immune system, create DNA, trigger enzymes and build proteins. It helps restore the skin's elasticity and contributes to a radiant glow. It also helps treat pores to reduce acne breakouts.

Foods that contain plenty of zinc include oysters, crab and other seafood, peanuts, lamb, dried watermelon seeds, roasted squash seeds, veal liver, whole wheat, roast beef, and toasted wheat germ.

2. Raspberries, blackberries and blueberries – These are fantastic sources of skin-healing phytochemicals and antioxidants, and of course, they are also quite delicious! You only need a handful a day to see results so start adding some to Smoothies or put them on your breakfast.

3. Green Tea – Rich in anti-inflammatory chemicals and antioxidants, green tea helps reduce soreness, redness and puffiness caused by acne. It also prevents potential acne breakouts. It's a wonderful detox for the body because it helps restore the skin and flush out infections. 3 cups of green tea is the equivalent of a cup of coffee as far as caffeine is concerned so start swapping it in your mornings for a caffeine hit that will do your skin wonders!

4. Whole grains – Fibre-rich whole grains like barley, oats, bread, pasta and cereal contain selenium, which is a chemical that helps stop inflammation and clear up acne.

5. Cucumber – It contains plenty of water component as well as fibre and vitamin C. It works best in cleansing your skin and getting rid of acne marks.

6. Coconut, Olive and Sesame Oil – These are excellent sources of monosaturated fats, which provide extra nourishment that your skin needs.

7. Natto (fermented soybeans) – Popularly eaten in Japan for breakfast, natto may taste a bit different and may also smell weird, but it does work wonders in getting rid of acne and skin blemishes.

8. Lemon Juice – Lemon is commonly applied to the skin as a natural method for lightening up the skin. Drinking lemon juice and other fruit juices will also help you have a healthier and blemish-free skin.

9. Yogurt – It's a probiotic that normalizes the digestive tract and helps control acne.

10. Salmon – Packed with omega-3 fatty acids, salmon helps in reducing skin inflammation and opening up clogged pores.

11. Purple and red foods – These include pomegranates, purple kale, acai, beets and other vermillion-coloured foods that contain antioxidants. They are great for rejuvenating the skin and preventing acne eruption.

12. Omega-3 fatty acids – Studies show that omega-3 fatty acids work great in reducing leukotriene B4 which is a major culprit in causing inflammatory acne. Take in an omega-3 supplement, or consume foods that contain omega-3 such as salmon, flaxseed oil, avocados and walnuts.

13. Coconut Water – This fun drink you would normally have when you are on an exotic holiday will also give you softer, brighter skin when consumed regularly. A glass of coconut water 3 times a week will give you noticeable nicer, softer skin all over. Add it to Smoothies and juices instead of water or have it by itself. Full of electrolytes this is a powerhouse drink of goodness.

Aside from the usual fruits and veggies, these are the top foods that can help ease your battle against acne. Try your best to incorporate a fair amount of these foods in your regular diet. You don't have to consume all of them simultaneously. The best approach is to set a specific meal plan that includes one or two anti-acne foods on a daily basis.

Foods to Avoid

If there are anti-acne foods that effectively nourish your skin and clear up acne marks, there are also those that serve to worsen acne breakouts. Stay away from junk foods, and minimize your consumption of the following:

1. Caffeine – Coffee and caffeinated black teas should be avoided as much as possible. Caffeine is a notorious trigger of acne mainly because it can cause hormonal imbalance and body stress. If you need something that will boost and revitalize your energy, go for coffee alternatives and healthy foods. Green Tea is the exception to this, so start swapping it with your current caffeinated drinks!

2. Sugar – Too much sugar can cause acne eruption due to an increase in insulin that leads to clogged pores. It's alright to consume sugary treats like chocolates but always keep in mind to take them in moderation.

3. Dairy – This includes cheese, milk and creamy desserts. Skin specialists believe that the sugar content and additives in dairy cause hormones to go off balance, hence leading to acne.

4. Oily and Fried Foods – Most of the items you order in a fast-food restaurant are terribly bad for your skin health considering that they are too oily, fried, salty or sugary. According to researchers, over-processed and low quality oils tend to raise insulin levels and clog up follicles.

5. Processed and Refined Foods – These foods contain high levels of salt, glutinous and glycaemic index. They promote build-up of bacteria that cause acne so try your best to avoid buying processed foods. Instead, focus on whole, organic and fresh foods especially green vegetables.

Changing your diet and replacing unhealthy foods with healthy ones may seem like a difficult task but your efforts will definitely pay off in the long run. You don't have to depend on skin care products solely when you can beautify and nourish your skin from the inside.

Make sure to have a varied and satisfying diet that contains a combination of fresh, organic items. Within a couple of weeks of consuming healthy meals, you'll surely notice a surprising difference in your complexion. Your skin will glow more radiantly with all the vitamins, enzymes, fibre and proteins that your everyday diet contains.

Chapter 2 Eliminating Acne by Changing Your Lifestyle

Now that you've learned about the best foods that are conducive to healthy, smooth skin, it's also time that you find out about the importance of having an anti-acne lifestyle. If you want to beat acne, you need to take better care of your skin every moment of the day. This involves not only skin care regimens but other valuable activities in your day-to-day life.

The top layer of your skin, called epidermis, is the largest organ of your body, and it's vulnerable to the environment around you. Your facial skin is particularly sensitive. The harmful UV rays, the dust and bacteria swarming everywhere, and your habits of touching and pinching your face are all contributing factors to acne breakouts.

Here are 10 lifestyle changes that will help you fight acne:

1. Get more sleep!

Have you noticed that you easily feel tired when you lack sleep? You might also notice more pimples and blackheads when you stay up late at night frequently.

Studies reveal that sleep deprivation is detrimental to the proper functioning of our body. It also greatly increases psychological stress which causes higher glucocorticoid production. What does this mean? It means that there's a higher risk for you to suffer from skin abnormalities and problems like acne. So, make sure to get enough sleep at night, preferably at least eight hours. And of course, maintain a regular sleeping cycle. Even if you sleep eight hours per day, sleeping at 2 am in the morning is still bad for your skin. Sleep as early as possible so you can also wake up early and start your day with a fresh, properly rested mind and body.

2. Exercise regularly.

Exercising is also crucial in keeping healthy skin. When you exercise, you'll not just get a physically fit figure (that of course helps boost your self-esteem and confidence tremendously); you'll also be able to battle acne effectively primarily because exercising the right way regulates hormone levels, strengthens the immune system and improves circulation of oxygen to skin cells, hence flushing out cellular wastes.

However, take note that uncomfortable sweating can possibly lead to acne eruption due to skin irritation so make sure to wear something comfy that allows your skin to emit sweat naturally. Also, take a shower afterwards to clean out all that sweat.

3. Drink plenty of water.

With adequate water intake, it's easier for your body to get rid of toxins and to hydrate your skin. It helps boost blood circulation to the skin. Water plays a critical role in eliminating waste materials from metabolism and lowering the level of toxins. To detoxify your body and prevent acne breakouts, make it a habit to drink lots of water every day.

4. Put on SPF before going out in the sun.

Slather enough SPF on your face before facing the harsh sunlight that contains harmful UV rays. Sunlight makes your skin dry. What's worse, your skin might get inflamed or burned, hence exacerbating acne pores and lesions that could lead to acne scars.

So, before heading outdoors, wear the right SPF for your skin. Choose products that are compatible with your skin type. If you have sensitive skin, go for lighter, non-clogging products with the "non comedogenic" label.

5. Cleanse your face twice a day.

Dermatologists confirm that there are more glands in the face that produce oils than any other body parts. On top of that, a concoction of makeup, dirt, dust and sweat clog up the pores of the face, inevitably resulting in acne. Always cleanse your face twice a day – once in the morning and once at night – to wash away all of these toxins. It's best to use non comedogenic products for a gentle cleansing regimen. Remember never to scrub your face when cleansing! Gentle, circular motions work well enough in washing away dirt. A good quality oil such as Olive oil or Coconut oil will remove your makeup without the need for a chemical makeup remover.

6. Exfoliate once or twice a week.

Bacteria tend to breed in dry skin with tiny cracks. Moreover, too much flaking leads to clogged pores. You can use a non comedogenic moisturizer after exfoliation.

Here are recommended natural ways to exfoliate your skin:

7. Sanitize your phone.

Did you know that your phone is a fertile breeding ground for germs? Thousands of bacteria stick to your mobile phone, quickly spreading to your fingers and your face via texting and talking. Wipe your phone with a bit of hand sanitizer at least once a day to keep it clean.

8. Apply hair products before washing your face.

Pomade acne typically occurs when hair products such as hairspray, gel, shampoo or conditioner cause acne breakouts. The oils from the products seep in the skin, thus trapping bacteria in the pores. To avoid this, try to apply the products before washing your face.

9. Avoid touching your face!

For some people, touching their face and squeezing tiny pimples have become unconscious habits that they just can't avoid. However, if you want to have a smooth and lovely skin, stop touching your face. Pay attention to those moments that you unnecessarily press your fingers on your face to feel a set of new, itchy pimples. Your fingers have countless dirt, bacteria, sweat and grime that are undoubtedly bad for acne. If you can't seem to change this habit, just try to wash your hands frequently.

10. Wash and change your fabrics.

Sheets, pillowcases, towels and clothes should be washed regularly to remove bacteria and oil.

Tip: Place a different, clean towel/cotton handkerchief on your pillow every night so your face doesn't come in contact with dirt and germs. You'll be surprised at how this works wonders in reducing acne.

11. Never sleep with makeup on.

It's a sure fire way to worsen your acne condition. Remove your makeup with a chemical-free makeup remover before rinsing with cleanser.

Chapter 3 Comprehensive Anti-Acne Skin Care Regimen

Find Out Your Type of Skin

We all have different types of skin. You might have an oily skin or a dry one. Also, you might either have a sensitive or normal skin. It's important to know your skin type because you may react differently to acne treatments and skin care products. Once you know your skin type, you can determine an ideal approach that works well to attain a healthier and smoother skin.

Read the different types of skin listed below, and find out the best anti-acne skin care regimen that suits yours.

Oily Skin – Oily skin shows large pores and appears shiny a couple of hours after cleansing. It's also vulnerable to whiteheads and blackheads. If you wear makeup, you may notice oil seeping through it most of the time. People who have oily skin are best recommended to choose oil-free face wash and non-comedogenic (non-clogging) products. You may also want to try salicylic acid as part of your treatment.

Cleansing: Use a cleansing bar for oily skin twice or thrice a day only. You may also use a gel cleanser as an alternative. Don't over-wash your skin because it can cause irritation.

Toning: It helps to use a salicylic acid treatment to lessen oil and maintain clear pores. Try applying a product with salicylic acid on your face, while focusing on the T-zone – nose, chin and forehead.

Moisturizing: An oil-free, non-clogging formula is preferable. Focus on drier areas and apply gently.

When putting on makeup, you can reduce the oily shine of your skin by using a water-based formula and paper face blotters. It also helps to use blotting powder and blush.

Dry Skin – Dry skin feels tighter and tends to be vulnerable to rough complexion. You may also develop wrinkles more easily. Cold weather tends to cause a flaky complexion. A gentle cleanser that doesn't remove the natural oils on your face is great to use. You should also add a moisturizing cream to your skin care regimen.

Keep in mind that scrubbing your face while washing or bathing can damage your skin so try to avoid it.

Cleansing tip: Use a cleansing bar or moisturizing cleanser with a soothing formula twice a day.

Toning: Skip this step if mild toners irritate your skin. If not, use a non-alcohol toner. Soak it in a cotton ball and glide gently over your skin.

Moisturizing: Instead of oil-free formulas, go for creamy ones. Alpha hydroxyl acid helps in exfoliating the skin. Products with panthenol, aloe or vitamin E help soothe the skin. Make sure to apply the moisturizing cream while your skin is damp but don't make it feel greasy. You should feel moist yet fresh afterwards. It's also good to apply a moisturizing mask one or two times in a week for exfoliation purposes.

For makeup: Use a moisturizing foundation for a smoother complexion.

Normal Skin – People with normal skin have cleaner complexion and barely visible pores. You may use a gentle cleanser for your face.

Cleansing: Wash your face with a non-drying cleansing bar two times a day.

Toning: A non-alcohol toner works effectively in toning a normal skin.

Moisturizing: Like the other skin types, oil-free lotion is highly preferable.

If you find blemishes on your skin, try using gel-based salicylic or benzoyl peroxide products. Don't forget to exfoliate once or twice a week with a non-drying mask.

Sensitive Skin – Fine pores are easily noticeable on people with sensitive skin. If you easily experience irritation and inflammation especially to cleansing and abruptly changing weather conditions, then your skin could be delicate and sensitive. You may also commonly experience red rashes during allergic reactions.

Use hypoallergenic products to take care of your skin. Test products first before applying them on your skin to ensure that they don't cause irritation. You can do this by dabbing a little bit of the cream or lotion in front of your ear, and wait for a day to see results. If your skin gets irritated, then discard the product immediately. Fragrance is usually harmful for your skin, including scented hair products, lotions and perfumes.

Cleansing: Choose a gentle, non-drying, fragrance-free, non-comedogenic lotion cleanser. Take note that scrubbing is a big no-no. Cleanse your face as gently as possible.

Toning: This isn't really good for your skin so you may want to skip this process.

Moisturizing: Go for fragrance-free, oil-free lotion specially formulated for sensitive skin.

Makeup: Use only fragrance-free and hypoallergenic makeup.

Combination – This type of skin is shiny, and prone to blackheads and unusually dilated pores. It can also be a combination of other skin types, sometimes being dry and flaky and other times oily. You'll notice oily nose and forehead areas, if you have this skin type. It's best recommended to use gentle and non-comedogenic cleansers as well as salicylic acid. Exfoliating the T-zone once or twice a week with a clay mask helps a lot in reducing acne breakouts.

Cleansing: Apply a mild, liquid cleanser twice or thrice a day.

Toning: Use salicylic acid astringent only on the chin, nose and forehead (T-zone). You can also use astringent pads.

Moisturizing: Choose non-comedogenic, oil-free formula, and focus on dry areas only.

Makeup: A shine-blotting, oil-free makeup is best applied on dry areas and the T-zone.

Extra Tips:

Avoid scrubbing! It will make your skin dry, blemished and irritated. It will also increase your risk of acne scarring and lead to worse breakouts. When applying cleanser or soap, wash your face in gentle, circular movements for a maximum time of one minute. Pat your skin dry afterwards with a clean washcloth instead of rubbing your face thoroughly.

Never over-wash because it will also cause a drier skin. Twice or thrice a day is enough to keep your skin clean and fresh.

Always check if the water is not too hot for you because hot water tends to over dry the skin. If you like to use warm water, make sure to test the water first with your hands.

Ensure that the washcloths and materials you use to clean up your face all completely clean. Use a soft cotton handkerchief for sensitive skin.

Wear sunscreen every time you go out, even during winter, because harmful UV rays can damage your skin throughout the year.

Know Your Type of Acne

Aside from finding out your skin type, it also helps to know what type of acne you have. It will guide you in sorting out and selecting acne treatments that are best suited for your type of acne. The more knowledgeable you are about your condition, the better you can make more informed decisions.

Inflammatory Acne

This results from the breakout of irritating substances around the follicle, as emitted by skin bacteria. When you have inflammatory acne, you'll most likely notice tiny pimples filled with pus. You'll also find cysts, nodules and papules. Topical treatment works great on inflammatory acne. You can use products containing salicylic acid, benzoyl peroxide and alpha hydroxy acid.

Hormonal Acne

This is caused by hormonal fluctuation. Most people who suffer from hormonal acne are teens, pregnant women and females in their periods. Hormones cause the oil glands to grow larger and produce too much oil, thus causing acne breakouts. Usually, you'll find hormonal acne on your chin, nose, forehead, neck, chest, shoulders and back. Topical treatments are good for treating hormonal acne. It's also essential to maintain a skin care routine and healthy diet.

Keep in mind that different skin types having varying skin care needs. There's no one-size-fits-all solution to treat all types of acne. Know your type of skin and acne so you can find the right skin care regimen and treatment that suits you well.

Steps involved in an anti-acne skin care habit:

1. Cleansing

2. Toning

3. Moisturizing

4. Masking

5. Exfoliating

As mentioned earlier, use gentle, non-clogging cleansers and moisturizers for acne-prone skin. A clay-based mask works great in drawing impurities from the skin's pores.

For treating acne, use products containing the following:

Benzoyl Peroxide – Lotions or soaps containing benzoyl peroxide effectively remove dead skin and quicken the cell regeneration process. When buying these products, choose those that comprise 3% or less benzoyl peroxide to avoid skin irritation.

Salicylic acid – This works great in sloughing off dead skin cells and promoting skin growth. Typically, it causes dry skin around the acne but it will dissipate later on once your skin regenerates.

Sulfur – Cleansers with sulfur also help eliminate acne. This chemical element is a natural remedy that effectively absorbs oil. It has anti-bacterial properties that get rid of trapped dirt in pores. It's great for treating red spots, clogged pores and inflammatory lesions. However, sulfur should be avoided if you have sensitive or dry skin.

Retinoid –Retinoid is well known as an anti-acne solution that cleans clogged pores and clears up the skin. It's a major ingredient in anti-aging products. It promotes collagen production and exfoliates dead skin cells to clear up the skin. It works best for getting rid of acne scars.

Azelaic Acid – Another anti-acne component is the antibacterial azelaic acid which reduces inflammation. This is recommended for acne that leaves dark spots on the skin.

Tea tree oil – This has similar benefits to benzoyl peroxide. It contains natural antiseptic qualities that destroy acne-causing bacteria. It also works safely on sensitive skin. Search for products containing less than 5% concentration.

Consistency Is the Key

Once you've found the right skin care regimen for your skin, be sure to maintain a consistent, daily routine. Make it a part of your everyday habits. In a few weeks, you'll definitely notice a huge difference on your complexion.

Chapter 4 3 DIY Facial Scrubs

Not sure where to start in cleaning your skin? Here are 3 super easy facial scrubs; these are yummy, so make sure to label them if you put them in the fridge!

1. Lavender and Oatmeal Face Scrub

This scrub has lovely lavender in it, so start by doing a tester with this one on your skin before you use it in case you have sensitivity to flowers. Otherwise you can use this one 3 times a week for great results!

This is a great Scrub to make a lot of leave in the fridge for next time.

Ingredients

1 Cup Lavender

½ cup dry lavender flowers, no stalks

½ cup powdered milk

2 teaspoons cornmeal

Combine all these ingredients in a bowl and massage into Damp skin, and then rinse it with warm water.

2. Olive Oil and Sugar Scrub

This is a great handy scrub, as generally the ingredients involved are always available in your kitchen! Also you can use this on your whole body by adding different types of sugar, coarser sugar for your body, finer if you like it gentler on your face!

Ingredients

1 Tablespoon sugar

1 Tablespoon virgin olive oil

Mix equal parts of olive oil and sugar to get a paste like consistency. Depending on the type of sugar, more or less oil may be required. Once mixed apply the mixture to your face or body and gently massage for a couple of minutes, and then rinse off with lukewarm water.

As this scrub has oil in it you may find after doing this scrub that your body already feels nice and moisturized, and so using moisturizer may not be necessary.

3. Strawberry and Honey Facial Scrub

This one is really yummy, and smells great! The honey is wonderful for soothing your skin and works as a natural moisturizer to it.

Ingredients

2 Tablespoons Honey

¼ cup mashed strawberries

Juice of 1 lemon

¼ cup yoghurt

Combine all these yummy kitchen ingredients in a bowl. Apply to damp skin, leave on for 10mins, and then massage in for the last minute before rinsing off with warm water. This is a mask and a scrub in one, as honey and yoghurt soothe and moisturise, while the strawberries and lemon help to clean the skin.

Chapter 5 15 Lush DIY Facial Masks

Wondering about natural facial masks that you can easily do at home? Here are fifteen lush facial mask recipes that can certainly make your skin smoother and lovelier. If you prefer to use natural ingredients that you can find in your kitchen, these facial masks are great solutions.

1. Aloe Vera Facial Mask

Aloe Vera contains niacin, vitamins and amino acids along with soothing, anti-inflammatory qualities. It helps make your skin look fresher, clearer and younger. Simply mix the following ingredients, and apply to your face for around 15-20 minutes. Wash your face with warm water afterwards, and then splash with cold water to close your pores. This gentle mask is best applied once a week.

Ingredients

6 tbsp of cucumber juice

2 tbsp of plain yogurt

4 tbsp of aloe Vera

2. Pumpkin Facial Mask

Pumpkin is rich in antioxidants that keep your skin young and fresh, and treats puffiness and redness. It also contains beta-carotene which protects the skin's collagen.

Ingredients

1/4 cup of pumpkin pulp

1 tbsp of honey

Mash the pumpkin pulp and maxi with honey. Damp your skin before applying, and leave the mask on for 15-20 minutes. Wash with water afterwards. You'll notice a softer and rejuvenated skin.

3. Cranberry Facial Mask

Cranberries are packed with ellagic acids which are antioxidants that help improve skin elasticity and also boost collagen production.

Ingredients

2 tbsp of crushed cranberries

1/4 cup of cornmeal

2 tsp of honey

1 tbsp of buttermilk

Mix all of these ingredients, and gently massage on your face for a few minutes. Wash with warm water afterwards.

4. Grape Facial Mask

Grapes are rich in antioxidants that help get rid of harmful free radicals. They also contain fructose that serve as moisturizing agents. This facial is generally good for all types of skin.

Ingredients

Several crushed red grapes

2 strawberries

1 pinch of flour

1 tbsp of honey

Upon crushing the grapes in a bowl, blend the flour, honey and strawberries to thicken the mixture. Apply on your face, and leave the mask on for around 10-20 minutes. Rinse with water afterwards.

5. Honey Apple Face Mask

Honey is such a beautiful thing to use on your face, and combined with either apple cider vinegar or lemon juice to cleanse the skin it is a great and easy face mask!

Ingredients

2 Tablespoons Honey

1 Tablespoon Apple Cider Vinegar or lemon juice

Combine both of these great ingredients in a bowl and then apply to a freshly cleaned face. Leave on for 20minutes, and then rinse off with luke warm water.

6. Papaya Face Mask

A really great and very easy face mask, this face mask has only 1 ingredient, Papaya!

Ingredients

1 slice of ripe Papaya with seeds and pulp removed

Remove the seeds and pulp for a piece of Papaya. Rub the inside of the papaya peel onto your skin after cleaning it. Focus on any problems area's such as wrinkles. Let it dry for 20min, and then rinse off.

7. Honey Facial

Very easy and no need to go to the supermarket, these ingredients are in the cupboard!

Ingredients

2 Tablespoons of honey

1 tablespoon of apple cider vinegar or lemon juice

Just combine the 2 ingredients together and apply generously all over your face. Allow to sit for 20min and then gently rinse off! So soothing!

8. Sour Cream Facemask

This one is very similar to the facemask above, but has the added ingredient of sour cream, this helps to heal scars, even out skin tone, exfoliate and brighten your skin all at the same time.

Ingredients

2 tablespoons sour cream

2 tablespoons honey

1 tablespoon apple cider vinegar or lemon juice

Combine all the ingredients together and apply all over a damp clean face, leave on for 20min, and then wash off with warm water.

9. Orange and Yoghurt Face Mask

For a revitalizing citrus facemask this facemask with yoghurt and orange is very refreshing!

Ingredients

1 tablespoon plain yoghurt

Juice from ¼ slice of orange

Some orange pulp

Teaspoon of aloe Vera

Combine these lovely ingredients together and leave on for at least 10minutes. Then gently rinse off and pat dry your face

Yoghurt is a lovely ingredient for a face mask, if you have no other ingredients just putting yoghurt on your face for 10-20min will help tighten pores and brighten your skin!

10. Avocado Face Mask

Avocado is such a great food and so good for your skin full of vitamins and minerals!

Ingredients

1/2 soft avocado

2 tbs hot water

1 teaspoon honey

Mash the Avocado with a fork in a small bowl. Dissolve the honey into the water and add it to the avocado. Gently apply to your face and leave on for minutes and wash away.

11. Honey and Coffee Facemask

Everyone loves there morning coffee, but did you know it's great for the skin too? Try this easy facial next time you are making your morning coffee.

Ingredients

1 Teaspoon used coffee grinds

Teaspoon of salt

Teaspoon of honey

Teaspoon of brown sugar

1 egg

Crack the egg into a small bowl and then combine all of the ingredients, the mixture should be thick and creamy. Apply to clean skin, and leave on long enough for the mask to harden. Then gently rinse off with warm water and pat dry.

12. Delicious Banana and Honey Mask

This is yummy, so try not to eat it whilst you are making it!

Ingredients:

1 ripe banana

1 teaspoon of honey

1 teaspoon of fresh lemon juice

Mask up the banana in a bowl and make sure to remove any chunks, mix in the honey and lemon juice. Apply to your face and leave on for 20min and then rinse off.

13. Egg Face Mask

Another facemask with fairly standard kitchen ingredients, grab this mask whenever you need some tightening up!

Ingredients

1/2 a lemon Juice

1 egg white

Beat the egg white and lemon juice for 3 min, and apply directly to your face, avoiding the eye area. Leave on for 30min and rinse off with warm water.

14. Green Tea Face Mask

Green tea isn't just good for your insides; it's also great for your skin.

Ingredients

Green tea

a tablespoon of granulated sugar

half a tablespoon of lemon juice

Make a cup of green tea with twice as much tea as you would normally have. Then either wait for the tea to cool down, or put it in the fridge until its cool. Take it out, mix in the sugar and lemon juice, pat it onto your face and either use it as a face wash or leave it on for 15 minutes. Wash off and pat dry.

15. Cucumber and milk Face Mask

What face mask list would be complete without a cucumber face mask!

Ingredients

1/2 cucumber

1/4 cup milk

1 tbsp honey

1 tbsp brown sugar

Mash or puree the cucumber. Make sure to remove any big bits, but before mashing save 2 round slithers for your eyes. Then combine the puréed cucumber with the rest of the ingredients, apply to your face, then apply the cumber pieces to your eyes sit back relax and was off after 20 min.

Chapter 6 Oil Pulling

Gargle the Oil in, Spit the Bacteria Out

People have always been on a quest to find the elixir of life. We've pretty much used everything to make ourselves look younger and more beautiful. From using conventional lotions and creams to using natural ingredients, we just keep on looking for more ways to get younger looking skin. We even resort to unorthodox practices that might look weird, but often end up getting the job done.

Oil pulling is one of those unorthodox practices. It is the process of gargling a teaspoon of oil. Yes, it sounds weird, but a lot of people vouch for it.

However, you might ask yourself this question – How could gargling oil help me have younger looking skin? The truth is, oil pulling wasn't intended to help the skin at all! Originally, people used oil pulling because of its oral-health benefits. It's been found out that the oil cleanses the mouth of bacteria and parasites. Moreover, people who use oil pulling reported having healthier gums and teeth. However, some realized that after a few tries, their skin suddenly became significantly healthier. It was then found out that oil pulling could help make people have healthier skin.

How does oil pulling help the skin?

The primary benefit of oil pulling is its ability to remove blemishes on the face. However, to understand how it prevents acne from growing, we have to first talk about how bacteria makes its way into the body.

Our mouths are the gateway to our body. When we eat something, everything ends up in our bloodstream, and then to our skin. Sometimes, however, some food remain in our mouth. When the leftovers deteriorate, bacteria proliferate. Although brushing our teeth helps reduce bacteria, some still make it through alive. Bad breath is one sign that your mouth still has bacteria. Having tonsillitis, on the other hand, suggests that the bacteria and parasites have infected your mouth.

As time passes, some of the bacteria and parasites are ingested into the body. Since these bacteria are unneeded by the body in the first place, the body tries to find a way to remove the bacteria. In the end, the bacteria makes its way to the skin. Most excess substances that can't be removed through defecation and urination are passed on to the skin. After the skin has reached a saturation point, it tries to remove the bacteria. Pimples and other blemishes simply mean that the skin is finding a way to clean itself. But we all know that pimples aren't as good as they sound. They're icky and just plain disgusting.

Oil pulling removes the possibility of acne from the onset because it cleanses the mouth of bacteria and parasites left by food. You don't need to worry about getting pimple outbreaks anymore. Some people even claim that oil pulling has helped them remove black heads and other skin defects. All in all, the detoxifying property of oil pulling leads to a blemish-free, glowing skin.

Oil pulling basics

By now, you must be hooked and eager to learn how to do oil pulling. The process is simple and only requires water, oil, and a lot of tolerance.

Firstly, you must clean your mouth and throat by drinking water. Now get a tablespoon of oil and swish it in your mouth. I would recommend a good quality Extra Virgin Cold Pressed Coconut Oil as the taste is a lot nicer or Extra Virgin Olive Oil. Be sure that it reaches every part of your mouth. The viscous texture of the oil makes it hard for bacteria and parasites to latch on the walls of the mouth. Bacteria then ends up in the oil. However, it takes a while to do all that. Although experts suggest newbies to swish for approximately five minutes, the average length of oil pulling is around 15 to 20 minutes. But anything is better than nothing, so if you need to start with 5minutes initially and build up then do it that way until you get to 15-20minutes.

After swishing, spit the oil out. Never swallow the oil because it contains all the bacteria within your mouth (you'd speed up the trip of the bacteria to the skin). Then, gargle your mouth with regular water. It might even be easier just to buy a second tooth brush just for oil pulling and give your mouth a brush with warm water after you do the oil pulling. This is too make sure that there is no oil left in your mouth. Finally, brush your teeth for a clean and white finish.

The drawbacks

Oil pulling might sound fine and dandy but it's a very tedious process. Not only does it require a lot of time to accomplish, it's also very challenging. The oil's viscosity makes it difficult to move it around the mouth. Moreover, oil isn't your usual mouthwash. Some people complain that oil is hard to gargle in their mouth. Others even say that it's downright uncomfortable. But with a little bit of practise this drawback is not a problem. If you wake up in the morning and stretch just put the oil into your mouth while stretching. If you can just slip Oil Pulling into your normal routine it will become very easy to form the habit of doing it daily!

Ways to make oil pulling better and tolerable

The best way to make oil's viscosity tolerable is to use different kinds of oil. The most commonly used variant is sesame oil or Coconut Oil. Some suggest olive and sunflower oils for newbies. Each kind of oil has a slightly different taste and texture. Try out different kinds of oil and decide which one you like best.

If oil pulling isn't really working out for you because of the texture, then you could opt to add another ingredient into the mix. Tea has been used to dilute the oil, thus making it less viscous.

Chapter 7 Clean Your Skin Like an Egyptian

Guasha: The Wonder Practice for Healthy Skin

A conventional skincare regime is expensive. Moreover, there isn't a guarantee that it'd work in the first place! If we could add up all of the expenses for skincare products, we'd notice that not only are they ineffective, but also costly. Imagine yourself buying lotions, creams, and astringents to get healthy skin, only to be dismayed at the results.

In the end, we realize that going back to basic natural practices, is the best way to care for our skin. One such way to get that young, glowing skin you've been dreaming of comes from a very unusual but very effective practice—guasha.

Guasha is an ancient practice that involves the use of paste made of baking soda and vodka. Yes, you've read it right, vodka can help you get healthier skin. The cleaning properties of the wonder powder (baking soda) is not only useful for teeth, but also for our skin. If these two could already do so much, what more if we use them together?

During ancient times, Egyptians took a bath in vodka-and-soda-powder paste. The Egyptians made vodka out of sugar, extracting its alcohol. They then mix it with sodium bicarbonate (baking soda) to make a slushy, yet coarse, paste. When the Romans came into Egypt, they were amazed at the glowing skin that Egyptians had. They were surprised that they managed to keep their skin smooth and healthy in spite of the scarcity of water. It should be noted that the Romans made sophisticated aqueducts and bath areas. Yet ironically, the water-deprived Egyptians have bested them in caring for the skin! Guasha eventually found its way into the modern world. Some people even prefer doing guasha every morning, rather than rely on conventional lotions and creams.

The wonders of guasha

Guasha can do a lot for the skin, from cleaning up pores to invigorating the skin cells. The vodka and the baking soda components of the guasha paste help each other out perfectly.

Scrubbing off dead skin cells

The skin is known to shed old cells as a way of maintaining itself. However, not all of the dead skin is taken out. Some are still left, which cause the skin to have a very dry texture. The baking soda within the guasha paste helps clear any leftover dead skin. Baking soda is a coarse substance. However, its rough texture isn't too rough that it would damage the skin.

Opens up pores

Once the skin is cleared of dead skin, the guasha paste could further use its coarse texture to open up the pores of the skin. Usually, the reason why people experience problems with their skin is because the pores are too clogged.

The skin is not only the biggest organ of our body, it's also the dirtiest. Our body relies on the skin pores to eject unnecessary toxins. However, when dead skin blocks the way of these pores, the body is unable to expel excess substances. Furthermore, having open pores makes it easier for the guasha paste to carry out its other functions.

Detox for the skin

After the pores open up, the guasha paste starts to clean the deep layers of the skin. Vodka kills bacteria and rids your body of toxins. The alcoholic content of vodka makes it easier for the body to detox the skin. If left alone, the toxins within the skin could prove to be harmful in the long run. Also, your skin will become prone to infections and diseases, if it's unable to clear out all the dirt (much more if the skin has clogged pores).

The acne prevention remedy

If the skin is filled with toxins, the body would surely find a way to expel all of those harmful substances. And what way could it be other than to make it ooze out of our pores. Acne is the result of our skin being saturated with toxins. The fluid within pimples is simply grime that the body has desperately tried to remove. Through guasha, the skin is cleansed of toxins that cause pimples, thus clearing our faces of any blemish. It's far better than using remedies that attempt to remove acne, because guasha prevents pimples from sprouting out in the first place!

Everyday Guasha

To start doing Guasha at home you will need some Baking Soda, some cheap triple distilled Vodka, and a Tupperware container. You want a container you can close so that you can keep the mixture handy if you don't use it all.

1/3 fill the Tupperware container with Baking Soda, then add another 3rd of the Vodka. Mix it all together and just add as much Vodka as you think you need from here, to make a paste like consistency. Generally 1 cup of the past mixture will be enough to wash the whole body of an adult. This is a very thorough way to clean the body and can be performed daily or a couple of times a week. If you are continually in an environment that would lead to unhappy skin, such as if you were to work in a kitchen where oil just ends up everywhere, you may find you need to do the process daily. But if for example you lead a fairly healthy lifestyle and work in a garden or stay at home you may find you only need to do it every few days. Just test the process out and find what works for you.

Guasha variants

Some have experimented with the basic guasha mix by adding more ingredients. You can add coconut milk to the guasha mix for a more soothing experience. Coconut milk is a primary ingredient in most lotions. Adding it to your mix is a perfect way to cap off your scrub. After cleansing your body inside and out, you can use coconut milk to add nutrients to your skin.

Others prefer to use tea as an additive (or as an alternative) to coconut milk. Tea has been known to detox the blood, and so it can aid vodka in cleaning the skin.

Or if you're a fan of having highly moisturised skin, but don't want to add a chemical to your body after doing Guasha put some good quality Oil, Olive Oil or Coconut Oil work well into the baking soda, Vodka mix. When you wash off the mixture some of the oil will have soaked in, leaving your skin soft and clean! Adding a little bit of oil is great for people with problems area's like dry feet and knees, or if you are in air-conditioning or heating all day which dry skin out in seconds.

Try and experiment by adding ingredients that have been proven to help clean the body. Find out for yourself what mix best fits your needs and expectations.

Chapter 8 Getting Rid of Acne Scars

Generally, there are two kinds of acne scars: raised and depressed. Raised acne scars show up above the skin's surface and usually cause painful itchiness and irritation. Depressed scars are those that appear as pits on the skin. Depressed scars can either be ice pick acne scars or rolling acne scars. The former refers to punctured marks on your skin while the latter refers to sharp scars. Hypertrophic scars appear thick and protuberant on the skin.

Acne scars are often tough to clear up, and they're undoubtedly frustrating to have on your face. You don't have to let those skin flaws ruin your confidence. Follow these methods to eliminate acne scars and brighten up your skin:

Topical treatments – If your scars are not hypertrophic ones, topical treatments may work well in removing them. Look for products that aim to promote collagen production. These products contain vitamin C, glycolic acid or AHA, and retinoic acid.

Lemon/Lime – Apply lemon or lime juice directly on the scars to lighten up the complexion.

Vinegar – Vinegar mildly removes the skin's top layer and promotes new skin cells.

Tea tree oil – This contains healing and soothing properties that make the skin smoother. However, this isn't a good solution for people with sensitive skin.

Rose water and sandal wood paste – Apply directly on the scars, and leave the paste on for 30 minutes to one hour. This natural remedy works great for people with sensitive skin.

Olive oil – Olive oil makes the skin soft and smooth. Massage the oil on the scars for several minutes every day.

If you'd like to try clinical treatments, microdermabrasion is best recommended particularly for atrophic scars. It buffs down the skin around your scar, evens out the surface and lessens the darkness of the scars. Another scar-removing method is chemical peel which removes the skin's top layer to allow skin regeneration. It helps get rid of scars without pigmentation. Make sure to visit a professional dermatologist to ensure a safe procedure.

Chapter 8 Controlling Your Stress Levels

Many people tend to experience more acne breakouts when they're stressed out and deprived of sleep. There are various stress behaviours that lead to bad skin: poor hygiene, poor diet, lack of exercise and constantly touching the face. The body also responds to stress in a way that's bad for the skin. When you're stressed out, your brain prompts the release of stress hormones such as cortisol. However, aside from experiencing a faster heart beat and sharper perception, you also get oilier skin.

Sebum – the oil that's produced in the hair follicle – travels upwards and takes dead skin cells along. It creates a protective coat once it gets to the surface. When too much sebum is produced, the pores of the skin become clogged, thus leading to acne breakouts.

As you can see, too much stress can only give you more acne. If you're constantly stressed out because of work and other problems, it's best that you engage yourself in fun activities and hobbies like sports and yoga. Find an interesting hobby that will soothe your mind and keep you busy. Don't keep hiding yourself in a comfort zone for a long time. It's best to go outdoors, frolic with friends and interact with people.

Try out a new activity that will give you a more positive outlook in life. Find time to relax and enjoy. The more optimistic you are, the better you can tackle your acne problems. Skin health is not just about physical and internal; it also involves mental and emotional health. When you believe that you can achieve a beautiful appearance, your body will work a way to meet with your goals more easily. On the other hand, if you always take a pessimistic approach, skin problems may only get worse in the long run.

People who suffer from acne experience stress along with low self-esteem and confidence. It's completely understandable knowing that acne can be a serious problem. However, now that you've understood a better, multifaceted approach towards beating acne, you should try to boost your confidence and improve your positivity.

Tell yourself that you can get rid of acne, and that you can overcome this obstacle in your life. Your mind is undoubtedly a powerful tool to get rid of acne. Always think of the best outcomes instead of worrying about the worst. Soon enough, with the help of a healthy diet, proper lifestyle, great skin care regimen, and excellent acne treatments, you can surely achieve a beautiful, smooth and radiant skin.

Steps to Success Action Plan

Steps to Success has been put together to give you somewhere to start on getting your skin gorgeous and healthy. Having glowing healthy skin, free from acne is the goal, and by starting with the activities listed here you will be well on your way to having beautiful clear skin!

To really have success you may need to use this action plan a few times and trial a few different things to get the result you're after. Test, Measure and Monitor needs to become your motto until you have beautiful clear glowing skin again.

Step 1- Read and understand about your type of skin and acne, without knowing this you wont really know where to start!

Step 2- Diagnose what type of skin you have

Step 3 –Decide what foods you could add to your diet straight away to start cleaning up our skin, and also what foods you could eliminate immediately for faster results!

Step 4- Take note of if you are stressed and how you could cut down on stress in your life!

Step 4 –Make a decision to do 2 facials a week, and 1 scrub.

Step 5.Test out the change in diet and lifestyle and doing facials for your skin for at least 3 weeks, after 3 weeks you should notice a difference in your skin looking and feeling clearer, younger and fresher. Make sure to take note of what each facial or scrub does to your skin, you may find lemon in any form is to drying for your skin, or using any oils is making your skin too oily. By taking notice of what works and feels best you will be much closer to having perfect skin.

Step 6- If the desired result has not been achieved please go back and see if there is anything else you could add to your diet to help you clear your skin. Have you managed to eliminate a lot of your stress? Re-evaluate what you have done so far and keep trying the yummy facials twice a week.

Step 7- How did you go with trying this new approach? Success? If not try another approach and see how you go. It may take 6 weeks before you find what works for you, or you may have success straight away, the thing to remember is that you don't have to have acne! You will find a way to get rid of it!

Beautiful Clear Skin is a lifelong dream, and can't be given up on easily. If you find the first couple of things you try don't work as well as expected, make some changes to what you are doing and try again! Having a healthy diet and lifestyle will certainly improve the quality of your skin, but making a commitment to living a healthier way is going to provide many more benefits, it is definitely something to strive for, and can change your life!

Conclusion

Thank you again for downloading this book!

I hope this book was able to help you to fully understand what type of skin you have, and what you can be doing to improve the quality of your skin and help illuminate some of that pesky acne! Having beautiful skin means having a healthy body and that is something to aim for!

The next step is to put this knowledge to good use and attempt to get the clear skin you have always dreamed off, you are off to a flying start by reading this book and taking advantage of the Action Plan included.

Finally, if you enjoyed this book, please take the time to share your thoughts and post a review on Amazon. It'd be greatly appreciated!

Thank you and good luck!

http://www.healthybodybooks.com

Bonus Chapter

This Bonus Chapter is from the book Grow Gorgeous Hair: The Most Effective Natural Solutions for Longer Healthier Hair! Enjoy!

Your Hair is What You Eat

As you may have observed from the previous chapters, it is important to keep a balanced diet to maintain a great hair. A balanced diet means the right amount of different food types that will suffice your body's recommended dietary allowances. Apart from the other food types, the most needed nutrition that your hair will need will be coming from protein sources. However, you will have to balance this with all other food types to ensure that you neither have the dry hair that lacks nutrition, nor the oily type. We will aim for a good balanced nutrition.

As mentioned, the hair is made up of 97% protein. This means that we will have to nourish it with a good supply of protein to ensure that it is kept healthy and well. Apart from protein, it needs a good supply of moisture as well to make it look healthy and flowing.

Here are some foods that can help us maintain our hair's good health.

Salmon. If you are not eating fish, then you better start doing so! Salmons are great sources of protein and vitamin D. These two elements are key to ensuring that the hair is not only kept healthy, but also strong and manageable. Apart from these two, it also has Omega-3 fatty acids that help our body make great hair. The same is found on the scalp and cell membranes of the skin. It helps maintain healthy hair and skin.

Walnuts. If eating fish really does not thrill you, then you can try eating this nut. This is also rich in Omega-3. Needless to say, the peanut family is a good source of protein, and walnuts are quite reliable in that field. Other nutrients found in walnuts include biotin and Vitamin D. These nutrients keep the hair's DNA from being damaged by the heat from the sun. Other scientists also say that it has a good and sufficient supply of copper that can make our hair look rich in colour.

Blueberries. Vitamin C is not only good for your immune system; it is also a key factor in blood circulation. Why do you need to have a good blood circulation for your healthy to be nice and shiny? Vitamin C ensures that there is a good circulation of nutrients in the scalp as well as the vessels supplying nutrients to the follicles. If follicles are fed nice, then the hair will surely love it.

Oysters. Zinc is a good nutrient that keeps the hair production stable. A loss of zinc in your body will discourage the body from creating hair, and will result to hair loss – including the eyelashes! It does not only have a good deal of zinc, it also has protein that, like what we learned earlier, and the hair is mostly composed of. A few ounces of Zinc translates to about four times of your body's daily protein needs.

Eggs. What could be the most practical source of protein other than eggs? Not only does it have protein, it also has all the other essential nutrients to hair growth. It has Zinc that is essential to hair production. Apart from that, eggs have a great supply of Iron that helps you move away from anaemia. Iron deficiency is the number one reason of hair loss, most especially in women. Getting a dose of eggs on a regular basis helps you achieve a great balanced diet; it also helps you achieve great hair and blood flow.

Sweet Potatoes. Probably now is a good time to love this if you're not fond of eating it. Sweet potatoes have a great deal of vitamin A. If you think Vitamin A is only good in keeping the eyes healthy and bright, it also gives our skin a boost of health, and keeps it away from being dry. Since our scalp is a skin, having a good supply of vitamin A prevents drying of the scalp. A dry scalp results to dandruff, so we must ensure a good supply of vitamin A at all times.

Milk and Cheese. Since the hair is 97% protein, we must find a conscious effort to ensuring that it is well fed at all times. Milk and cheese, being products from animals, are good sources of protein. It also contains iron, which we learned earlier to be a key ingredient in hair production, as well as Zinc.

Other types of food that you should consciously manage to eat regularly are those rich in fibre and vitamins. A good supply of fruits and cereals will do the trick. While fibre does not directly affect hair production, you need to ensure that your body is scraped-off with toxins on a daily basis. Fibre cleanses the body with unwanted toxins and keeps our digestive system healthy at all times.

Your hair will get a hefty deal of proteins with the suggested food mentioned earlier. Try adding them on your salads, or slowly introducing them to your daily diet. Eight glasses of water a day will ensure that your body is properly hydrated as well. 3% of the moisture that your hair will require will be coming from the water you take in so ensure that there is sufficient supply of water in your body.

Apart from your hair, eating these nutritious foods and getting them included on your daily diet will also benefit you skin. In fact, it is possible that the first effects are seen on your skin first prior to seeing them on your hair. Apart from your skin and you hair, your body as a whole will be affected by your improved dietary practices. A healthy body is the best "side-effect" that improving your hair quality may cause. It is just like hitting two-birds in one stone!

www.ingramcontent.com/pod-product-compliance
Lightning Source LLC
Chambersburg PA
CBHW020940160726

47993CB00007B/2856